Paleo Recipes With Slow Cooker

Enjoy Your Paleo Dishes Without The Work

Kevin M. White

Contents

Chapter One

Introduction

I'd like to thank you for downloading Paleo Slow Cooker Cookbook: Top 80 Paleo Recipes - Easy, Delicious, and Nutritious Paleo Diet Cooking, and I'd want to commend you on it.

For health-conscious people all throughout the world, the Paleo diet is the go-to abstention from food. It's a diet that encourages people to choose more traditional food kinds as the foundation of their diets. While some go full out and accept every single food item, the majority choose for a more relaxed version of the diet that just restricts the intake of unusual foods.

However, because of the difficulty of preparing the Paleo diet or other weight-loss strategies, a large number of individuals seem to avoid them. After a long day at work, it's incredibly tempting to just order in or have your dinner delivered. I know what you're going through since I've been in your shoes.

When I get home from work, making dinner is the first thing on my mind after an 8-hour shift and a couple of other extended periods of unplanned spare time.

My response is the slow cooker or stewing pot, which is often overlooked yet very essential. This fantastic kitchen is back, and rightfully so! Consider preparing a reliable and tasty recipe that will take 10 hours to prepare while you sleep. That's a possibility with the slow cooker! I can't tell you how many times I've woken up to a delicious supper that was still hot from the oven, as if I had just finished preparing it.

Begin your journey to a healthier and more efficient lifestyle by following the Paleo diet with your slow cooker. This book has more than 75 plans.

This book's plans are divided into four categories:

Recipes for Beef

Recipes for Chicken

Recipes for Seafood 16

Recipes for 16 Vegetables

Breakfast, sides, and desserts are available in 16 different combinations.

Once again, thank you for downloading this book; I hope you like it!

Beef Recipes, Chapter 1

4 Servings of Beef with Broccoli 1 pound chuck roast, 1 pound brisket, 1 pound brisket, 1 pound

florets from 3 cups broccoli

sliced and cored apple

12 cup stock (beef) raw honey (third cup)

coconut aminos (around 1/3 cup) 3-garlic cloves

Apple and garlic should be placed in a slow cooker.

Stock, honey, and coconut aminos are added to the slow cooker. In a slow cooker, add the meat and stir to combine.

Cook for 5 hours on low with the lid off. Remove the lid and add the florets of broccoli. Cook for 30 minutes more, covered.

Serve

Beef Stroganoff is a dish that is prepared using beef. 6 servings beef stew meat (pounds)

8 ounces sliced mushrooms

12 sliced onion

1 tblsp. powdered garlic 1 tblsp. powdered onion paprika, 2 tblsp.

a quarter teaspoon of thyme

coconut cream, 1/3 cup

red wine vinegar, 1 tsp to taste with salt and pepper Direction:

Garlic powder, onion powder, paprika, and thyme should all be blended in a mixing basin before being left away.

Place the meat in a mixing dish and season it with the spice combination.

Set aside after mixing until the meat is well covered.

In a slow cooker saucepan, place the onion and mushrooms.

Arrange the meat so that the coating-covered side is on top.

Cook for 4 to 12 hours on low, covered.

Remove the lid and stir in the coconut cream and vinegar. Toss in a pinch of salt and pepper to taste, and mix to combine.

Serve Title: Beef Meatballs Cook for a further hour on low heat, covered.

2 servings + 1 pound ground beef

6 zoodles

14 cup chopped spinach 2 tbsp finely diced onion

1 teaspoon of extra virgin olive oil

1 cup sauce for spaghetti

To taste, add salt and pepper.

Clean the zucchini under running water before preparing the spaghetti.

Using a mandolin slicer, thinly slice the zucchini. Fill the colander halfway with noodles.

Allow for 5 minutes of rest and drying after sprinkling salt on the surface.

Fill a pot with water and add the noodles.

Bring water to a boil, then remove from the heat and put aside for 2 minutes.

Put the beef, onion, spinach, and garlic in a mixing dish to make the meatballs.

Salt & pepper to taste.

If required, use your hands to completely blend the ingredients. Make balls out of the meat mixture and place them in a pan.

Cook meatballs in a hot pan until both sides are golden.

Place the meatballs in the bottom of the slow cooker pot and pour your favorite sauce on top.

Cook for 5 hours on low with the lid off. On a platter, arrange the spaghetti.

The meatballs and sauce should be on top. Serve

6   PALEO RECIPES WITH SLOW COOKER

4 servings of Spicy Beef beef chuck (pounds) 3-garlic cloves 1 shallot

2 c. coconut milk (full-fat) curry powder, 2 tblsp

12 tbsp chile sauce 12 ginger, peeled

to taste with salt and pepper Cut the meat into tiny pieces according to the directions.

Set aside the meat cubes in a slow cooker saucepan.

In a food processor, combine the onion, garlic, and ginger and pulse until a paste-like texture is achieved.

Cook for 3 minutes with onion paste in a saucepan.

Allow to boil for another 8 minutes with the coconut milk. Sprinkle curry powder, salt, and pepper over the mixture in the slow cooker pot. Mix in the chili sauce until it's completely smooth. Cook for 20 minutes with the lid closed.

Cook for another 20 minutes after removing the lid. Serve

Rosemary Beef Stew

6 people 2 pounds beef stew meat 1 pound ground beef

carrots (1 pound)

an 8-ounce glass cranberries radishes, 2 bunch 2 onions and 1 pound celery root

garlic, 2 cloves

fresh rosemary, 2 sprigs 3 cup broth (bones)

to taste with salt and pepper Fill a slow cooker halfway with meat, carrots, and celery root.

Pour the broth in a bowl and season with salt and pepper to taste. Blend until smooth.

Place 2 onions in the pot's center and arrange the garlic cloves on top. Top the cloves with rosemary. Cook for 8 hours on low with the lid off.

Take the sprigs from the cover and toss them out. In a blender, combine the garlic cloves and onions. Take

2 ladles of liquid, blended

Puree in a food processor until smooth.

Refill the slow cooker with onion purees. Stir in the cranberries

Cook for 30 minutes more, covered. As required, add salt.

Serve

12 servings of beef and chili Ingredients:

1 pound of cubed beef stew meat

28 oz tomato puree 1 pound ground beef cup beef broth

12 c. pureed pumpkin

2 cups mushroom slices 1 zucchini squash, chopped

6 garlic cloves, minced 1 onion, chopped 1 tblsp. powdered garlic

chile powder (about 3 tbsp) cumin 1 tbsp

olive oil, 1 tbsp

Cook the meat until it is browned in a skillet.

Cook until the zucchini squash is tender, then add the olive oil, mushrooms, and garlic. In a slow cooker saucepan, combine the broth, pumpkin puree, tomato puree, garlic powder, chili powder, and cumin; mix well and put aside.

Set aside the slow cooker pot with the vegetables.

Combine the olive oil and chili powder in the same pan and stir thoroughly.

Cook until both sides of the beef stew meat are brown, while covering it with the chili mixture. Simmer for 2 hours on high, then reduce to low and cook for another 5 hours.

kg flank steak Ingredients: Ropa Vieja Servings: 8

14 cup extra virgin extra virgin extra virgin extra virgin extra virgin extra virgin extra virgin extra

14 cup chopped cilantro 2 garlic cloves (minced)

14 cup parsley, coarsely chopped 1 tablespoon balsamic vinegar Tomato paste (12 oz.)

garlic powder (1 tbsp) oregano, 1 tbsp

cumin powder (1 tblsp)

1 tbsp flakes de onion coconut oil, 2 tblsp

to taste with salt and pepper Steak should be thinly sliced.

Cook half of the steak strips in coconut oil in a skillet. Each side should be cooked for 2 minutes.

Half-cooked

In a slow cooker pot, combine the cooked steak strips with the remaining ingredients. In the slow cooker pot, stir until everything is well combined, using your hands if necessary.

Cook for 6 hours on low with the lid off. Take the strips by removing the cover. Re-mix after shredding

Serve

'Pulled Beef,' as the name suggests, is a dish that 6 people
Ingredients:

14 cup veggie stock 3.5 lbs pot roast Tomato paste, 2 tbsp

tsp garlic (12 tblsp)

paprika (14 tbsp)

a quarter teaspoon of cinnamon

oregano, 12 tbsp

12 tblsp chile ancho

cumin (12 tsp) Sauce recipe

a third of a cup of stock that has been skimmed garlic, 2 cloves

14 diced onion

14 tsp chile ancho

12 CUP SARANGER

a quarter teaspoon of cumin

diced jalapeos

to taste with salt and pepper Pour stock into a slow cooker pot for the beef, then add tomato paste and gently stir to combine.

Put oregano, cumin, cinnamon, paprika, and ancho chile in a pot roast and season with oregano, cumin, cinnamon, and paprika.

To taste, season with salt and pepper.

5 hours on high, covered

Using forks, shred the meat from the slow cooker. Take

Remove the meat juices from the pot and set them aside in the fridge.

When the fat has solidified, remove it from the surface and pour the meat juice into a saucepan for the sauce. Add the jalapeno, garlic, and onion to a medium-sized skillet over medium heat. Cook for 5 minutes on low heat.

Combine the salsa, tomato, cumin, and ancho chile in a mixing bowl. Salt & pepper to taste.

Pour over shredded beef, stirring gently. Serve

Beef Brisket with Cabbage is a dish made with beef brisket.

6 people 1 pound corned beef brisket Ingredients: 1 pound beef brisket

onion

1 gallon of beef broth a stalk of celery

1 spud

cabbage, 1 head

avocado oil (about 1 tbsp)

to taste with salt and pepper Prepare the celery stalk, carrot, and onion by chopping them coarsely. Put everything in the slow cooker. Pour the broth over the noodles. Top the vegetable pieces with beef brisket.

Set aside for 6 hours on low after covering and cooking for 6 hours on low. Preheat the oven to 450 degrees Fahrenheit (230 degrees Fahrenheit).

Make 8 wedges out of the cabbage head. Place on a baking sheet and bake

Oil-based glaze

Season to taste with salt and pepper. Cook for 25 minutes in the oven

Serve the beef brisket with a side of cabbage. Beef Bourgignon is a type of beef.

Ingredients: pound beef stew (servings: 6)

2 peeled, sliced carrots 1 rutabaga 1 rutabaga rutabaga rut

2 tbsp tapioca starch 2 cups bone broth 12 lb sliced mushrooms

2 garlic cloves (minced)

rosemary (2 sprigs)

2 tsp mustard (Dijon) 14 cup red wine vinegar 1 onion (chopped) 2 leaves of bay

water, 2 tbsp

to taste with salt and pepper

Season the meat liberally with salt and pepper.

Cook until the meat is golden brown on all sides in a pan with coconut oil. Remove the meat and any juices from it, and replace it with the garlic and onion.

Cook, stirring frequently, until the onion is translucent. Pour

Mustard, vinegar, and broth Allow to simmer, then return the meat to the pan with the juices. Fill slow cooker halfway with meat and broth.

Mushrooms, rosemary, bay leaves, rutabaga, and carrots should all be added to the pot. Remove the cover and cook on low for 8 hours. Remove a ladleful of the liquid and pour it into a saucepan. Heat until it boils.

Tapioca and water should be combined in a mixing bowl. Fill a saucepan halfway with the tapioca mixture. Whisk the sauce until it thickens, about 5 minutes.

Pour the sauce into the slow cooker and stir everything together until everything is well combined. Take out the rosemary and bay leaves.

Braised Beef with Olives is a delicious appetizer.

4 people 2 pound chuck roast of beef

olives (15)

1 pound of thinly sliced carrots

garlic cloves, chopped

12 c. chopped leeks

12 tbsp olive oil 12 tbsp basil sprigs thyme

arrowroot (12 tbsp.)

water (1/4 cup)

to taste with salt and pepper Fill a small bowl halfway with the mixture. 2 garlic cloves, basil, 1 tablespoon olive oil, and 1 teaspoon salt, mixed well Set aside after rubbing the spice all over the roast. Place the remaining oil in the slow cooker, turn it up to high, and sear the meat.

Beef should be eliminated.

Cook for 4 minutes with the remaining garlic and leeks Season with salt and pepper and add the carrots and thyme.

Water should be poured.

Carrots should be topped with meat.

Cook for 6 hours on low with the lid off. Remove the cover and the meat from the pan. Place the carrots in a bowl and shred them with a fork.

Remove the liquid from the pot and stir in the arrowroot until the mixture thickens. Fill a plate with beef. Pour sauce on top. Serve with extra virgin olive oil on the side.

Servings: 6 Ingredients: Beef Pot Roast

Beef roast, 2 pound

Cremini mushrooms (eight ounces)

4 halved carrots garlic, 2 cloves

1 shallot

1 gallon of beef broth

celery seed, 12 tsp

12 tbsp parsley (dried)

to taste with salt and pepper Fill a slow cooker halfway with beef stock and set it aside.

Season the roast with celery seed, salt, and pepper. Place the roast in a slow cooker

Carrots should be added to the roasting pan and arranged around it. Onions, sliced, should be placed on top of the roast.

Cook on low heat for 7 hours.

mushrooms as a cover

Cook for 1 hour more with the lid on.

Borscht Ingredients: 1 pound beef stew meat, 8 servings

chunky potatoes

2 carrots, peeled and chopped into small pieces 4 chopped beets

cabbage, 1 head

1 shallot

Garlic, 4 cloves 28 oz tomatoes, diced 2 cup beef broth Tomato paste (six ounces)

parsley, 1 tsp

bay leaf (one)

1 tblsp dill (optional)

red wine vinegar, 6 tblsp

to taste with salt and pepper Put the beef stew meat, tomatoes, potatoes, beets, carrots, and onion into the slow cooker. Combine the tomato paste, broth, vinegar, parsley, dill, and salt and pepper in a mixing bowl and stir to combine. Fill the slow cooker halfway with broth.

Remove the cover and cook on low for 9 hours.

Serve Title: Beef Ribs Cover and cook for another 30 minutes on high 2 pound beef ribs, 4 servings

a chopped onion

1 crushed garlic clove

a tbsp grass-fed butter red curry paste (2 tbsp) Put in the pan as directed. 1 tbsp. margarine

Cook until the beef ribs are browned. Cook the cooked ribs in a slow cooker.

Combine the paste, onion, garlic, and the rest of the butter in a mixing bowl. Beef Broth Title: Beef Broth Cooking Instructions: Cover and cook on low for 8 hours. 4 quarts of beef bones Ingredients:

1 onion, chopped 2 carrots, chopped 2 celery stalks, chopped 7 garlic cloves, chopped 2 leaves of bay

Carrots, celery, garlic, and onion should be placed in a slow cooker with salt.

Bay leaves and salt are added to the bones. Add vinegar to the mix.

Pour enough water to completely submerge the bones. Cook for 10 hours on low with the lid off.

Remove the cover and strain the liquid.

Store

4 servings Beef and Balsamic Vinegar

carrots, halved

3 cut-up sweet potatoes 1 gallon of beef broth

2 garlic cloves, chopped rosemary sprigs 2

chopped onion

Leaves of bay

balsamic vinegar (about a third of a cup) coconut oil, 2 tblsp

to taste with salt and pepper Set aside the beef chuck roast after seasoning it with salt and pepper on all sides.

Beef chuck roast is cooked in coconut oil in a skillet.

Cook for 3 minutes on each side, until golden brown.

Cook the cooked chuck roast in the slow cooker.

Garlic, leaves, sprigs, and onion should all be added at this point. Add beef stock to the pot.

Cook for 6 hours on low with the cover off, then add the potatoes and carrots. Cook for an additional 3 hours, covered.

Remove the bay leaves and rosemary sprigs from the pot and discard the cover. Fill a saucepan halfway with the liquid from the slow cooker.

Bring to a boil until the sauce is the desired consistency. Refill the slow cooker with the sauce. Stir until the beef is completely covered in the sauce. Serve

Chicken Recipes, Chapter 2

4 Servings Title: Bacon and Chicken Ingredients:

5 breasts de chicken olive oil, 5 tbsp ten slices bacon

thyme, 2 tbsp

1 tbsp (one tablespoon) rosemary

oregano, 1 tbsp

salt, 1 tbsp Fill a slow cooker pot halfway with chicken breasts and bacon slices. Drizzle

using extra virgin olive oil

Spices and salt to taste

Remove the cover and cook on low for 8 hours.

a fork into the chicken meat Olive oil should be drizzled on top. Serve

Jerky made from chicken 4 people Whole chicken, cut into large chunks is one of the ingredients.

1 tsp powdered onion 2 teaspoon powdered garlic cayenne pepper (1 teaspoon) white pepper, 2 tsp

paprika, 4 tblsp.

a quarter teaspoon of salt

black pepper, 1 tsp Directions: In a large mixing bowl, combine onion powder, garlic powder, cayenne pepper, white pepper, paprika, salt, and black pepper.

Using running water, wash the chicken.

Using a paper towel, lightly dry the meat before placing it in the bowl.

Make sure all sides of the meat are well coated with the spices.

In a slow cooker pot, place the rubbed chicken.

Cook for 6 hours on low with the lid off.

Using a fork, shred half of the chicken pieces. Half of the plate should be boned.

On the other side of the plate, spread the shredded cheese.

Soup with Tortillas de Pollo de Pollo de Pollo de Pollo de Pollo de Poll

6 people Skinned and cut into thin strips chicken breasts 1

chopped onion

2 cups shredded carrots 28 oz diced tomatoes 4 cloves garlic, minced

32 oz chicken broth jalapenos, seeds removed and diced 2 cups celery, chopped bunch cilantro, chopped Tomato paste, 2 tbsp

1 tablespoon cumin 1 tablespoon chili powder 2 c.

olive oil, 1 tbsp

to taste with salt and pepper

In a slow cooker pot, pour the olive oil.

14 cup broth, garlic, onions, and jalapeno pepper Salt & pepper to taste.

Chapter Two

Cook, covered, on low heat until onions are soft

Cook for 2 hours on low with the lid off. Using a fork, shred the chicken. cilantro sprigs Serve

6 servings Chicken Cacciatore Ingredients: 1 pound chicken thighs

crimini mushrooms (eight ounces)

plum tomatoes, whole, 28 oz 14 cup whole wheat flour and 2 onions 14 cup white wine, 1 celery rib a sprig of rosemary

salt, 2 tsp

12 tblsp. cayenne Using running water, clean the chicken.

Sprinkle salt and pepper over the chicken in the slow cooker pot. Remove the stems and quarter the mushrooms.

Remove the celery's top and bottom ends. Cut an onion in half vertically.

Fill the slow cooker halfway with mushrooms, celery, and onion. Combine the tomatoes, flour, and white wine in a large mixing bowl.

Cook 4 hours on high, covered.

Lemongrass-Spiced Chicken Drumsticks

10 skinned chicken drumsticks (servings: 4)

lemongrass stalks

1 onion, 14 cup scallions

ginger, 1 tblsp

1 garlic clove (minced) 4 garlic cloves

coconut milk, one cup

coconut aminos, 3 tblsp 2 tbsp tamari

a tsp of spice

to taste with salt and pepper Directions: Season the drumsticks with salt and pepper and place them in a bowl. Pulse milk, fish sauce, coconut aminos, ginger, garlic, and spice powder until smooth in a blender.

Fill the bowl with the milk mixture and the chicken.

Combine onions, drumsticks, and marinade in a slow cooker pot. Cook for 5 hours on low with the lid off. Serve with a sprig of scallions on top.

Fajitas de Pollo con Pollo de Pollo de Pollo de Pollo de Poll 4 people 14 oz diced tomatoes 1 onion, thinly sliced 1 pound deboned and skinned chicken breast

2 cups thinly sliced bell peppers

12 tsp cumin 1 tsp oregano 4 cloves garlic, minced

12 teaspoon chili powder with chipotle 1 tsp coriander seeds

to taste with salt and pepper Step 1: Place the chicken breasts in a slow cooker pot.

Bell pepper, garlic, and onion go on top of the chicken.

Cumin, coriander, oregano, chili powder, and salt and pepper are sprinkled on top.

Tomatoes are poured

Cook for 6 hours on low with the lid off. Using a fork, shred the chicken. Serve

Stroganoff with Chicken

8 people Ingredients:

2 pound cut-in-thirds chicken hearts pound

quartered mushrooms (slices) 1 shallot Garlic, 4 cloves

Greek yogurt (7 ounces) 1

1 cup stock made from chicken

14 cup coconut milk (about) 1 tsp mustard (Dijon)

12 tablespoons cayenne

paprika (12 tblsp)

to taste with salt and pepper Place the mushrooms and onions in the slow cooker pot.

Add the heart of chicken.

Garlic, mustard, and the rest of the spices should be added at this point. Pour the stock from the chicken.

Cook for 6 hours on low with the lid off.

Allow 5 minutes after removing the lid. Combine the yogurt and cream in a bowl.

Allow another 10 minutes to settle after stirring. Thai Chicken Soup is a dish that may be served as a starter or as a main 10 servings

1 chicken breast, entire

1 lemongrass stalk, cut into big chunks ginger (5 slices)

lime (one)

20 leaves basil

to taste with salt and pepper Place the entire chicken, half of the basil leaves, lemongrass, ginger, salt, and pepper in the slow cooker.

Fill to the top with water.

Cover and simmer on low for 10 hours. Scoop into a serving dish and stir with the lime juice. Toss basil leaves in a bowl with a little olive oil and a pinch

Serve

Curry with Chicken 4 people 2 pound chicken breasts, chunked 14

coconut milk (ounces)

1 cup tomato juice 1 cup tomato paste 1 cup tomato paste 1 cup tomato paste 1 cup tomato

1 c. chopped broccoli

1 cup sliced carrots 1 cup chopped green beans

1 c. chopped onions

1 tbsp cinnamon 1 cup chopped tomatoes 1 cup chopped red bell pepper

a teaspoon of cumin and a teaspoon of garlic powder a tsp of ginger powder

2 tblsp coriander, ground 1 quart of liquid

To taste, season with salt Place the chicken and veggies into a slow cooker pot.

Combine the tomatoes and milk in a mixing bowl and whisk to combine.

Combine the ginger, cinnamon, coriander, ginger, and garlic in a large mixing bowl.

Stir with some water.

Sprinkle with salt and cook on low for 8 hours.

Artichokes de Poulet de Poulet de Poulet de Poulet de Poulet de Poulet de

8 people Ingredients:

2 entire chickens chopped into big chunks for the chicken ghee, 2 tblsp

1 shallot

Garlic, 4 cloves

lemon juice (14 cup)

2 cups stock made from chickens to taste with salt and pepper Spices are used.

14 tblsp cinnamon powder

12 tblsp cumin powder

tsp turmeric (12 tblsp.)

garam masala (1 tsp)

a quarter teaspoon of ginger powder

12 tsp flakes de pimentón

to taste with salt and pepper a cup of caperberries as an add-on

lemons

2 washed and drained cans of artichoke hearts 2 tblsp flour de tapioca

parsley, 2 tbsp

water, 2 tbsp Directions: Combine the spice ingredients in a mixing basin and stir until smooth. Set aside. Clean and dry the chicken pieces.

Salt & pepper to taste.

Cook for 5 minutes in ghee in a skillet with chicken. In a slow cooker, place cooked chicken.

Cook for 3 minutes in a pan with the garlic and onions

Combine the chicken stock, spice mix, lemon zest, and lemon juice in a large mixing bowl.

Simmer for a few minutes before pouring into the slow cooker vessel.

Cook for 6 hours on high with the lid closed.

Caperberries, lemons, and artichoke hearts are all good additions to this dish. Cook for an additional 1 hour, covered.

Remove the lid from the pan and combine the chicken, caperberries, lemon slices, and hearts in a mixing bowl.

Fill a strainer halfway with the liquid in the slow cooker. Fill a pot halfway with filtered liquid.

In a saucepan, combine 2 tablespoons water and the tapioca flour. While stirring, cook for 1 minute.

Over the chicken bowl, pour the sauce. Serve

Chili made with chicken. 10 portions Ingredients:

28 oz crushed tomatoes 15 oz tomato sauce 2 pounds ground chicken

1 onion (diced) 14 oz tomatoes

3 tbsp. garlic

1 tblsp. powdered onion 2

cumin (1 tsp)

oregano, 1 tbsp

chile powder (about 3 tbsp) basil, 1 tbsp

cayenne pepper, 12 tsp

1 pound diced carrots 1 minced jalapeo 1 c. diced celery

1 pound chopped red bell pepper

1 tblsp. chopped green bell pepper

To taste, add salt and pepper.

Add garlic and onions to a pot. Cook until the chicken is brown, about 5 minutes.

Fill the slow cooker halfway with the cooked chicken mixture. Red and green bell peppers should be added at this point.

Celery, carrots, and jalapeño peppers should be added at this point. Toss in the tomatoes, diced and smashed. Tomato sauce should be added.

Combine the spices, cayenne pepper, chili powder, cumin, basil, oregano, onion powder, and salt and pepper in a small mixing bowl. In a slow cooker, sprinkle Stir everything together well.

Cook on low heat for 6 hours.

6 servings Title: Garlic Wings 3 pound chicken wings 1 pound sour cream

tbsp cayenne pepper, minced tbsp garlic olive oil, 2 tbsp

honey (34 cup)

to taste with salt and pepper Chicken wings should be placed in a slow cooker.

Garlic, cayenne pepper, olive oil, and honey in a mixing bowl Salt & pepper to taste. Blend until smooth.

Fill slow cooker with mixture. Cook on low heat for 6 hours.

Servings: 4 Chicken, Vegetables, and Coconut 1 pound deboned and skinned chicken thighs

corn for baby

peas (cup)

coconut milk (1 cup) quartered onion

Garlic, 4 cloves

2 tablespoons minced ginger butter, 2 tbsp

1 teaspoon of extra virgin olive oil 1 tsp ground turmeric, 2 tbsp arrowroot 1 tblsp. cumin powder

1 tsp coriander, ground

to taste with salt and pepper Cumin, turmeric, coriander, salt, and pepper should all be mixed together in a small basin. Pulse onion, garlic, and ginger until smooth in a food processor.

Butter should be added to the slow cooker

Cook for 2 minutes on high, stirring after each addition.

Cook for a further 2 minutes, stirring occasionally. Pour milk over the chicken and place it in the slow cooker. Corn cobs should also be included.

Cook for 4 hours on low, covered. Stir in the arrowroot.

Cook for 30 minutes more with the peas. Serve

4 Servings Title: Cashew Chicken a pound of deboned and skinned chicken thighs, cut into bite-size pieces

12 cup toasted cashews 2

coconut aminos tbsp ghee 2 onions and 2 tablespoons rice wine vinegar

1 tbsp sesame oil 3 garlic cloves tbsp palm sugar

paleo ketchup (around a tablespoon)

12 tsp flakes de pimentón

arrowroot powder (1/4 cup)

To taste, add salt and pepper.

Flour and pepper should be placed in a bag.

Shake the bag to coat the chicken.

Cook the chicken in ghee in a skillet

With the exception of the cashews, combine all of the ingredients in a mixing bowl. Place chicken and sauce in a slow cooker.

Cashews are an excellent addition.

Serve Title: Chicken Masala Cover and cook on low for 3 hours

4 servings 1 pound deboned and skinned chicken thighs

1 cup coconut milk 1 cup onion, sliced garlic, minced

2 quarts crushed tomatoes 1 tsp coriander seeds

14 teaspoon chili powder 1 tablespoon minced ginger garam masala (2 tbsp) 1 tblsp. cumin powder ghee, 2 tblsp

1 tablespoon palm sugar

1 tbsp garam masala, 1 tbsp ghee, 1 tbsp ghee, 1 tbsp ghee

Brown the chicken thighs in 1 tbsp ghee in a pan. Cook the chicken in a slow cooker.

Cook garlic and ginger in the remaining ghee in a pan Tomatoes and milk

Cumin, flakes, sugar, salt, and the rest of the masala should be sprinkled on top. Simmer for a while

Fill slow cooker with mixture. Cook for 3 hours on low with the lid off. Serve

Chicken Cheese and Chili is the name of a dish made up of chicken, cheese, and

4 people 1 pound of deboned and skinned chicken breasts

a chopped avocado

2 minced garlic cloves 1 cup salsa bell peppers

chopped onions

1 minced jalapeo

1 tblsp cayenne pepper 1 cup water 1 tablespoon cumin

to taste with salt and pepper Chicken, cumin, chili powder, onion, garlic, and water should all be placed in a slow cooker.

Salt & pepper to taste. Remove the cover and cook the chicken breasts on low for 8 hours. Shred the cabbage with a fork.

Place the meat in the slow cooker again.

Cook for 5 minutes in a skillet with the jalapeo and peppers. In a slow cooker, combine jalapeno and pepper.

Cook for 20 minutes after stirring. Place on a plate and top with avocado. Serve

Seafood Recipes (Chapter 3)

6 servings of Shrimp Curry 1 pound cooked, tail-off shrimp 1

400ml coconut milk 1 cup chicken broth lemongrass, 1 bunch a teaspoon of ginger powder cilantro, 1 tblsp

a quarter teaspoon of ginger powder

lemon juice (14 cup) Step 1: Place the shrimp in a slow cooker. Pour

milk, broth, and lemon juice Sprinkle

spices with lemongrass Cook for 2 hours on high, covered, until ready to serve.

Salmon Soup (servings: 4)

Noodles made from zucchinis 1 tbsp ginger, minced 1 green garlic, minced 1 onion, sliced

coconut aminos (1/4 cup)

14 cup vinegar (coconut) chives (1 tsp)

1 tablespoon chili powder Put the salmon, ginger, and garlic in the slow cooker.

Until the fish is completely submerged in water, pour water. Cook 2 hours on high, covered.

Remove the cover and remove the fish, as well as any bones from the fish.

Return the fish meat to the slow cooker, along with the strained broth.

In a slow cooker, combine the minced ginger, onions, garlic, coconut vinegar, and coconut amino

Cook for 20 minutes on low heat with the lid off.

Take off the cover and stir in the zucchini noodles.

Cook for 15 minutes more, covered. Into bowls, ladle soup Chives and chilies should be added at the end. Tilapia with Honey on the Side

4 tilapia fillets Ingredients:

10 oz mandarin oranges, peeled and drained 1 tbsp honey balsamic vinegar, 2 tablespoons

Directions: Lay aluminum foil on a flat surface and season with salt and pepper to taste.

Place the fillets in the foil's middle.

Over the fillets, drizzle honey and vinegar. a few orange slices on top

With the foil, fold and seal the fillets. Foils should be placed in a slow cooker.

Cook 2 hours on high, covered.

Salt and pepper the foil after opening it. Serve

Jambalaya de Shrimp

4 people

Ingredients:

2 cup Andouille sausage 1 pound deveined shrimp 1 cauliflower head 4 ounces chicken meat 5 cup stock made from chicken

3 tbsp. Cajun seasoning 3 onion cloves, diced

4 oz. chopped red bell peppers

14 cup aioli 2

bay leaf Place chicken, garlic, onions, peppers, Cajun seasoning, bay leaf, and hot sauce in a slow cooker.

Pour the stock from the chicken.

Cook for 5 12 hours on low with the lid off. Remove the lid and add the sausages to the pan. Cook for another ten minutes, covered.

Cauliflower should be cut into small pieces and placed in a food processor.

until the rice has reached the desired texture

Remove the lid and add the cauliflower and shrimp to the pan. Cook for 20 minutes more with the lid on. Chowder de Pescado de Pescado

Ingredients: Ingredients: Ingredients: Ingredients: Ingredients: Ingredients: Ingredients

3 pound dory (cream) Turnips, 20 small

2 c. carrots, small 2 squashes yellow

chicken broth (64 ounces) coconut milk (two cans)

8 crumbled slices of bacon 1 shallot

2 tblsp. minced garlic celery, 2 pieces

1 tbsp. cayenne

COOK, COVERED, ON LOW HEAT UNTIL ONIONS ARE SOBT

to taste with salt and pepper Cut the fish into cubes according to the recipe's instructions. Fill slow cooker halfway with water. chicken broth with cubed fish

Place vegetables in slow cooker, cut into small pieces. Stir in the bacon, garlic, and red pepper.

Remove the cover and cook on low for 10 hours. Stir in a pinch of salt and pepper.

Salmon and Spinach Platter (Servings: 4) 4 salmon fillets Ingredients:

2 cup spinach 4 cup spinach

2 lemons 1 tablespoon dill

12 cup white wine (approximately)

to taste with salt and pepper Fill a slow cooker halfway with spinach and top with salmon fillets.

Dill, salt, and pepper are sprinkled on top.

1 lemon, sliced into wedges, should be placed on top of the fillets. Wine should be poured.

Cook for 2 hours on low with the lid off.

Remove from the oven and place on a plate

wedges from the rest of the lemon Over the fillet, place the wedges on top. Serve

Glazed Salmon is the name of the dish. 4 people Ingredients:

2 fillets de saumon

1 tblsp mustard (Dijon) olive oil, 2 tbsp

a teaspoon of ginger powder honey 3 tbsp

1 tsp crushed red pepper Mix mustard, oil, ginger, honey, and flakes together in a mixing bowl until well combined.

Put into parchment packet the salmon

In the packet, add the mustard glaze. In a slow cooker, place the packets. Cook for 2 hours on low with the lid off.

Serve

Spicy Salmon Mustard is a name for a dish made with a spicy salmon and

2 people 2 garlic cloves and salmon fillets 1 teaspoon of extra virgin olive oil

a couple of tablespoons Mustard de Dijon

1 tsp cayenne pepper 14 tsp cayenne pepper cayenne pepper cayenne pepper cayenne pepper ca

grated ginger tbsp Put all of the ingredients in a mixing bowl.

Toss the salmon in the dressing to coat all sides. Fill a parchment bag halfway with the fillets.

COOK, COVERED, ON LOW HEAT UNTIL ONIONS ARE SOFT

Chapter Three

Pour the stock from the chicken

Cook for 5 12 hours on low with the lid off. Remove the lid and add the sausages to the pan. Cook for another ten minutes, covered.

Cauliflower should be cut into small pieces and placed in a food processor.

until the rice has reached the desired texture

Remove the lid and add the cauliflower and shrimp to the pan. Cook for 20 minutes more with the lid on. Chowder de Pescado de Pescado

Ingredients: Ingredients: Ingredients: Ingredients: Ingredients: Ingredients: Ingredients

3 pound dory (cream) Turnips, 20 small

2 c. carrots, small 2 squashes yellow

chicken broth (64 ounces) coconut milk (two cans)

8 crumbled slices of bacon 1 shallot

2 tblsp. minced garlic celery, 2 pieces

1 tbsp. cayenne

to taste with salt and pepper Cut the fish into cubes according to the recipe's instructions. Fill slow cooker halfway with water. chicken broth with cubed fish

Place vegetables in slow cooker, cut into small pieces. Stir in the bacon, garlic, and red pepper.

Remove the cover and cook on low for 10 hours. Stir in a pinch of salt and pepper.

Salmon and Spinach Platter (Servings: 4) 4 salmon fillets Ingredients:

2 cup spinach 4 cup spinach

2 lemons 1 tablespoon dill

12 cup white wine (approximately)

to taste with salt and pepper Fill a slow cooker halfway with spinach and top with salmon fillets.

Dill, salt, and pepper are sprinkled on top.

1 lemon, sliced into wedges, should be placed on top of the fillets. Wine should be poured.

Cook for 2 hours on low with the lid off.

Remove from the oven and place on a plate

wedges from the rest of the lemon Over the fillet, place the wedges on top. Serve

Glazed Salmon is the name of the dish. 4 people Ingredients:

2 fillets de saumon

1 tblsp mustard (Dijon) olive oil, 2 tbsp

a teaspoon of ginger powder honey 3 tbsp

1 tsp crushed red pepper Mix mustard, oil, ginger, honey, and flakes together in a mixing bowl until well combined.

Put into parchment packet the salmon

In the packet, add the mustard glaze. In a slow cooker, place the packets. Cook for 2 hours on low with the lid off.

Serve

Spicy Salmon Mustard is a name for a dish made with a spicy salmon and

2 people 2 garlic cloves and salmon fillets 1 teaspoon of extra virgin olive oil

a couple of tablespoons Mustard de Dijon

1 tsp cayenne pepper 14 tsp cayenne pepper cayenne pepper cayenne pepper cayenne pepper ca

grated ginger tbsp Put all of the ingredients in a mixing bowl.

Toss the salmon in the dressing to coat all sides. Fill a parchment bag halfway with the fillets.

In a slow cooker, place the bag

Cook for 3 hours on low with the lid off. Remove parchment from the oven.

Serve

Servings: 4 Ingredients: Seafood Asparagus Title:

four fillets of tilapia

asparagus (1 bunch) lemon juice (12 tbsp) butter, 2 tbsp

1 teaspoon of black pepper Place one fillet at a time on an aluminum foil-covered flat surface.

Arrange the asparagus on top of the fillets in an even layer. Drizzle lemon juice over the butter.

Seal the folds.

Place all of the fillets in foil-lined slow cooker. Cook 2 hours on high, covered.

Serve

6 servings of Shrimp Tacos Ingredients:

11 oz peeled shrimp 12 cup chopped red bell pepper 14 oz diced roasted tomatoes

salsa

1 tblsp minced garlic

cumin (12 tsp)

12 tsp cayenne olive oil, 2 tbsp

6 taco shells 4 tablespoons cilantro

to taste with salt and pepper Put shrimp in a slow cooker and cook on low for a few hours.

1 tbsp olive oil drizzled on top Sprinkle salt and pepper over shrimp Toss in the tomatoes and herbs.

Mix in 2 tablespoons cilantro.

Cover and cook on low for 4 hours.

Rest of the cilantro on top. Set aside the taco shell. Fish and Cilantro as a Side Dish

Ingredients: Ingredients for 6 servings: Ingredients for 1 serving: Ingredients for 1 serving

six fillets of tilapia

12 tsp minced garlic 1 tsp dried cilantro lime juice, 2 tblsp Taco shells sprinkled with salt

Fillets should be placed in the slow cooker. Combine cilantro, garlic, lemon juice, and salt in a large mixing bowl. Remove the cover and shred the fish with a fork after 4 hours on low. Fill shells with the scoop.

Serve

4 servings of fish with parsley 2 pound cod fillet 1 cup sour cream

lemon

1 piece of fruit

12 oz.

4 tablespoons of extra virgin olive oil parsley, 2 tbsp

to taste with salt and pepper Place the fish fillets in the slow cooker. Over the fillet, scatter the remaining ingredients. Cook for 2 hours on low with the lid off. Serve

Mussels' name 4 people 2 pound mussels 8 ounces mushrooms diced 28 ounces tomatoes diced 4 garlic cloves minced 3 shallots diced 2 tablespoons oregano

basil, 1 tbsp

paprika, 1 tblsp.

3 tsp red chili flakes 1 tsp red chili flakes 1 tsp red chili flakes

olive oil, 1 tbsp

to taste with salt and pepper Place the olive oil in a pan.

Garlic, mushrooms, and shallots should all be added at this point.

Cook until golden brown, then transfer to the slow cooker.

In a slow cooker, combine all of the ingredients except the mussels. Cook for 5 hours on low with the lid off.

Take the cover off the pot and add the mussels.

Cook for 30 minutes on high, covered, before serving.

6 servings of Crab Chowder 12 cup sweet corn kernels 12 oz crabmeat 4 cup broth de poulet

butter (tbsp)

1 smashed potato

1 shallot

chilies, 4 oz.

thyme (12 tsp)

12 teaspoon paste de chili

seasonings Directions: Melt butter in a pan and sauté onions until they are translucent. Place all ingredients in a slow cooker. Remove cover and puree mixture with a hand blender for 8 hours on low. Serve

Cioppino is a dish that is served with a tomato sauce. 8 people Ingredients:

1 pound mussels, 1 pound cubed tilapia, 1 pound clams

12 Crab Meat (Cooked)

1 pound crushed tomatoes 28 oz

8 oz tomato paste (chopped onion) white wine, 1 cup

4 tbsp parsley green pepper, chopped

oregano, 1 tsp

a quarter teaspoon of thyme

basil tsp

1 tblsp. chili powder

1 teaspoon cayenne

seasoning with salt and pepper to taste

All ingredients, except the seafood, should be placed in a slow cooker. Cover and cook on low for 8 hours, stirring occasionally. Cover and cook on high for 30 minutes, stirring occasionally. Salmon with Cranberries as a Side Dish

4 salmon fillets Ingredients:

12 cup dried cranberries 1 cup chicken broth 12 cup dried cranberries 1 cup butternut squash, seeded and cubed

a quarter teaspoon of thyme

olive oil, 1 tbsp

to taste with salt and pepper Place the cranberries and squash into the slow cooker.

Pour the broth over the noodles.

Salt & pepper to taste.

Cook on low for 5 hours. Remove the cover and gently mash the mixture.

In the slow cooker's pot, evenly distribute the mixture. Fillets should be well coated in thyme, salt, and pepper. Olive oil should be used to coat the surface.

Fillets should be placed in a slow cooker

Cook for an additional 25 minutes on low heat, covered.

Serve

Vegetable Recipes (Chapter 4)

4 Servings of Split Pea Soup Ingredients:

2 cups rinsed split peas 1 cup split peas 1 cup split peas 1 cup split peas

2 garlic cloves, chopped 12 tsp rosemary carrots, chopped cup celery, chopped 1 onion tbsp parsley, chopped 1 bay leaf 2 tsp basil dried

water (four cups)

to taste with salt and pepper Split peas, onion, celery, carrots, cloves, basil, rosemary, and basil should all be placed in the slow cooker.

Cook for 10 hours on low with the lid off.

Fill bowls with mixture.

Add parsley to finish

Serve

Veggie Korma is a dish that can be made with a variety of vegetables. Ingredients: Ingredients: Ingredients: Ingredients: Ingredients: ingredients: ingredients: ingredients:

florets of cauliflower, cut 2 chopped carrots 1 cup green beans

garlic cloves, minced 12 cup green peas 2 tbsp curry powder 1 onion (chopped) almond meal, 2 tblsp coconut milk, 1 can

to taste with salt and pepper Cauliflower, green beans, carrots, green peas, garlic, and onion should all be mixed together in a slow cooker.

Curry powder and coconut milk should be combined in a bowl.

Mix in the salt until it's evenly distributed.

Fill the slow cooker halfway with milk.

Almond meal, if desired.

Cook for 8 hours on low, covered, before serving.

Soup with Mixed Vegetables is a dish that can be made with a variety of vegetables.

8 people 6 red potatoes, cubed 1 onion, diced 1 pint grape tomatoes, halved 1 head celery, diced 2 tsp garlic powder chicken broth (32 oz.)

to taste with salt and pepper Potatoes, celery, onion, and carrots should be placed in a slow cooker. Chicken broth should be poured in.

Garlic powder, salt, and pepper are sprinkled on top of the dish.

Fill slow cooker pot halfway with water and cook on low for 30 minutes.

Remove the cover and toss in the tomatoes and kale. Cook for an additional 10 minutes on low heat, covered. Serve

6 servings of pumpkin curry 15 ounces coconut milk 1 cup pumpkin puree 1 cup stock made from vegetables

3 thinly sliced carrots 12 tbsp curry powder 3 cups sweet potatoes, cubed 1 chopped onion

14 tsp turmeric powder 1 garlic clove (minced) garam masala, 2 tsp lime (one)

to taste with salt and pepper Pour pumpkin puree and vegetable stock into a slow cooker. Garam masala, turmeric powder, curry powder, salt, and pepper are sprinkled over the dish.

Blend until smooth.

Mix in the potatoes, carrots, onion, lime juice, and garlic until everything is thoroughly combined. Cook for 6 hours on low with the lid off.

Serve

4 servings of Vegetarian Stew Ingredients:

12 head cabbage, chopped 3 cups shredded carrots 2 zucchini, chopped 1 head celery, chopped

1 shallot

chicken broth (32 oz.)

minced garlic cloves (5 cloves)

2 jalapeo peppers, seeded and finely chopped chili powder (1 tbsp) cumin 1 tbsp

1 c. chopped cilantro 2 tablespoons olive oil 2 tablespoons tomato paste 2 c.

to taste with salt and pepper Directions: Pour broth and olive oil into a slow cooker. Add jalapeno, onions, garlic, salt, and pepper to taste. Cook on low heat, covered, until the vegetables are soft.

Remove the cover and stir in the rest of the ingredients. Fill the pot halfway with water and cook on low for 2 hours.

Cauliflower, Garlic, and Dill is the name of a dish made up of three ingredients: cauliflower, garlic, and d

4 people Cauliflower, head 6 garlic cloves 1/3 cup dill (chopped)

a tablespoon of coconut milk and a pinch of salt

to taste with salt and pepper Cauliflower should be placed in a slow cooker.

Leaves and stems should be sliced on the bottom. florets from the head

Half of the dill and garlic should be added at this point.

Fill the cauliflower with water. Cook for 8 hours on low with the lid off.

Drain liquid into a colander after removing the lid.

Remove the dill and place the cauliflower and garlic in a mixing bowl. Salt & pepper to taste.

Pour the milk into a bowl and stir in the dill. Blend the mixture.

Pulse until you achieve the desired texture. Serve

Minestrone Soup is a soup that is rich in vegetables.

6 people Ingredients:

2 cups diced carrots

chopped shallots

28 oz tomatoes, diced 28 oz veggie broth tsp cayenne pepper 1 tsp basil 1 cup spinach, chopped 2 stalks celery, diced

oregano, 1 tsp

parsley (tsp)

Leaves of bay

olive oil, 2 tbsp

to taste with salt and pepper Step 1: Pour the olive oil into the slow cooker.

Celery, carrots, potatoes, zucchini, garlic, and shallots should all be added at this point.

Chapter Four

Pour veggie broth and tomatoes with juice

Add spinach

Sprinkle parsley, basil, oregano, cayenne and salt Stir

and add bay leaves

Cover and cook for 8 hours on low Remove cover and discard bay leaves Serve

Title: Summer Veggies

6 people Ingredients:

2 cups zucchini, sliced 1 cup mushroom, sliced 2 cups okra, sliced

1 cup grape tomatoes

½ cup olive oil

½ cup balsamic vinegar 1 tbsp thyme, chopped 2 tbsp basil, chopped

1 cup onion, chopped

To taste, add salt and pepper.

Put in a bowl zucchini, mushroom, okra and tomatoes, toss and set aside

Put in another bowl olive oil and vinegar, stir

Add into vinegar mixture thyme and basil Put into slow cooker tossed veggies Drizzle with the vinegar mixture

Toss until all veggies are coated with the marinade Cover and cook for 3 hours on high, stir every hour Serve

Title: Kale and Red Pepper Frittata Servings: 6 Ingredients: 5 oz kale oz feta, crumbled 8 eggs oz red pepper, roasted 2 tsp olive oil

¼ cup onion, sliced

½ tsp all purpose seasoning blend

to taste with salt and pepper Direction:

Clean kale and dry with paper towels

Put into slow cooker the olive oil

Set to low and cook kale for 4 minutes Chop peppers slice onions

Add to slow cooker

Beat eggs and pour into slow cooker Stir everything together well. Sprinkle with feta, salt and pepper

Cover and cook for 3 hours on low Serve

Title: Squash Soup 6 people Ingredients: 6 cups butternut squash, chopped 2

carrots, chopped 2 apples, cored and chopped 1 clove garlic, chopped

chopped onions

cups veggie stock

½ tsp sage

1 cup almond milk

thyme (12 tsp)

1 tbsp parsley, minced

to taste with salt and pepper Direction: Put into slow cooker, squash, carrots, apples, garlic and onion

Pour stock

Sprinkle sage and thyme

Cover and cook for 8 hours on low Remove cover and pour milk, stir

Pour contents to blender and pulse until smooth Sprinkle with parsley, salt and pepper to taste Serve

Title: Mashed Cauliflower and Garlic

6 people Ingredients: 1 head cauliflower 1

tbsp sage, minced

1 tbsp thyme, minced

1 tbsp rosemary, minced 1

tbsp parsley, minced 1 cup vegetable broth 3 tbs ghee

6 cloves garlic

6 cups water

to taste with salt and pepper Direction: Remove leaves from cauliflower head and cut into florets Put

into slow cooker florets and garlic

Pour broth and then water to cover the florets Cover and cook for 6 hours on low Remove cover and drain the liquid Put cauliflower back into slow cooker Add ghee and mash with hand blender

Add sage, thyme, rosemary and parsley Sprinkle salt and pepper to taste Mix and keep warm Serve

Title: Carrot Soup Ingredients: Ingredients for 6 servings: Ingredients for 1 serving: Ingredients for 1 serving

2 carrots, chopped

1 lb cauliflower onion, chopped 3 cup veggie stock

½ cup coconut milk a chopped onion

cloves garlic, chopped

to taste with salt and pepper Direction: Put into slow cooker garlic, onion, cauliflower and carrots

Pour stock Cover and cook for 6 hours on low Add salt and pepper

Pour milk

Use hand blender and pulse until smooth Serve

Title: Apple and Ginger Soup

4 people Ingredients:

2 apples

1 butternut squash, cubed 3 cups veggie stock 14 oz coconut milk

¼ tsp nutmeg

1 tsp curry powder

1 tbsp ground ginger 1 shallot

to taste with salt and pepper Direction: Put into slow cooker all ingredients except milk Cover

and cook for 8 hours on low

Pour into blender and pulse until smooth Add milk and pulse again

Serve

Title: Tomato Puree Servings: 4 Ingredients: 3 tomatoes, chopped

a chopped onion

8 cloves garlic, minced

¼ cup cilantro

¼ cup green pepper

1 tsp balsamic vinegar

To taste, add salt and pepper.

Put into slow cooker tomatoes and use hand blender to make it smooth

Put into pan onion and garlic, cook until clear Add into slow cooker with rest of ingredients Use blender and pulse again until smooth Cover and cook for 4 hours on low

Serve

Title: Cashew Curry Servings: 4 Ingredients:

1 cup cashews

1 butternut squash, cubed 14

coconut milk (ounces)

1 tbsp curry powder 1 tbsp ginger, grated

cumin (12 tsp)

½ tsp red chili paste

3 cloves garlic, minced 1 onion, cut into chunks lime (one)

to taste with salt and pepper Direction: Pour milk into slow cooker

Add ginger and garlic

Juice the lime and pour into slow cooker Add spices, stir until well combined Add onions and squash Cover and cook f0r 6 hours on low Serve

Title: Hazelnut Puree

Servings: 4 Ingredients: 1/8 cup hazelnuts

5 parsnips

2 apples

4 cups veggie stock

½ cup half and half cream a chopped onion

½ tsp ground cardamom

to taste with salt and pepper Direction: Preheat oven to 400 degrees

Put parsnips, onions and apple into oven and roast for 30 minutes, set aside when done

Pour veggie stock into slow cooker

Sprinkle salt, pepper and cardamom Add roasted apples, onions and parsnips Cover and cook for 6 hours on low Use a hand blender and pulse until smooth Add half and half cream

Hazelnuts should be sprinkled on top.

Serve

Soup with Sweet Potatoes

4 people 3 pound sweet potatoes, peeled and diced

5 cup vegetarian stock 2 carrots, diced 2 celery stalks, sliced 1 onion, chopped 1 garlic clove, minced

coconut milk (1 cup) Salt

to taste with salt and pepper Put potatoes, carrots, celery, onion, garlic, and vegetable stock in a slow cooker.

Season with salt and pepper and cover.

and cook on low for 6 hours

Remove the lid and combine with a handheld blender until smooth. Pour in the coconut milk and whisk well.

Cook for another 30 minutes, covered. Serve

Recipes for Breakfasts, Sides, and Snacks (Chapter 5)

Breakfast Casserole is a recipe for a breakfast casserole.

6 people

a dozen eggs

1 pound of beef sausage

1 cup shredded sweet potato 1 cup sliced leeks 1 cup chopped kale 2 tsp garlic 2 tbsp coconut oil

to taste with salt and pepper Directions: Melt coconut oil in a skillet.

Chapter Five

Cook until the kale, garlic, and leek are aromatic

Combine the egg, sausage, sweet potato, and sautéed kale combination in a mixing bowl. Fill slow cooker halfway with water. Cook for 6 hours on low with the lid off.

Applesauce Ingredients: 1 jar Title: Applesauce Servings: 1 jar

6 pound apples

4 sprigs cinnamon

a teaspoon of vanilla Peel the apples, core them, then cut them into smaller pieces. Put the apples, sticks, and vanilla in the slow cooker. Top and simmer on low for 6 hours. Remove the cover and toss out the cinnamon sticks. Refrigerate the mixture after mashing it and putting it in a jar. Serve

4 servings of potato mash Ingredients: 1 pound sweet potatoes

1 tsp nutmeg powder

1 tbsp cinnamon powder

14 tsp cloves (ground)

12 teaspoon allspice

1 quart of apple juice

to taste with salt and pepper Potatoes should be peeled and sliced into small pieces.

Fill slow cooker halfway with water. 12 cup apple juice should be poured

Garnish with cinnamon, cloves, nutmeg, and allspice. Cook for 5 hours on low with the lid off.

Remove the lid and combine with a hand blender. While adding the remaining apple juice, pulse. Serve

Breakfast with Sausage

10 portions

1 pound sausage

12 oz cheddar cheese, shredded 6 russet potatoes, shredded 12 eggs, whisked

6 chopped onions

4 tbsp unsalted butter, melted

to taste with salt and pepper Directions: Place shredded potatoes in a slow cooker.

Pour the melted butter into the pan and season with salt and pepper. Toss until everything is properly blended.

Slice the sausage into tiny pieces. Arrange the sausage slices on top of the potatoes. Pour eggs into a bowl. grate some cheese

Cook for 8 hours on low with the lid off. Place onions on the plate's side.

Serve

6 servings Title: Fig Butter 20 stemmed and halved dried figs 1

1 apple cider cup

12 c. honey

3 apples, cored and diced 6 apples, cored and diced

a teaspoon of cinnamon

14 teaspoon nutmeg

12 tsp cloves (ground) Salt Directions: Combine figs and apples in a slow cooker.

Combine apple cider and honey in a mixing bowl.

Cinnamon, nutmeg, cloves, and salt are sprinkled on top. Lid and simmer on low for 8 hours. Remove cover and transfer to food processor. Pulse until completely smooth.

Refrigerate after storing in a jar. Serve

Paleo Oatmeal Serving Size: 2 Ingredients: 2 cubed apples

1 diced butternut squash

12 c. almonds

12 c. walnuts

1 tbsp sugar (coconut) coconut milk (1 cup) 1 teaspoon of cinnamon

12 teaspoon nutmeg

Prepare nuts ahead of time by placing almonds and walnuts in a basin and submerging them in water.

Soak for 12 hours with salt. Rinse well under running water.

Put everything in a food processor.

Pulse until the texture is grounded.

Put apples, squash, nutmeg, cinnamon, sugar, milk, and ground almond and walnuts in a slow cooker.

Cook for 8 hours on low, covered, before serving.

4 servings Mexican Casserole Ingredients: 8 eggs

12 pound cooked and shredded bacon 1 cubed potato

1 chopped bell pepper

8 oz. chopped mushrooms

to taste with salt and pepper In a skillet, sauté the onions until they are tender.

Bacon, bell pepper, potato, onions, mushrooms, and eggs go into the slow cooker.

Stir everything together well.

Salt & pepper to taste. Cook for 8 hours on low, covered, before serving.

Breakfast Pie is a recipe for a breakfast pie. 6 people Ingredients:

a dozen eggs

1 pound sausage, peeled and chopped into little pieces 1 shredded sweet yam

1 chopped onion

garlic powder (1 tbsp) 2 teaspoon basil

1 tablespoon of coconut oil

to taste with salt and pepper Directions: Grease the surface of the slow cooker with coconut oil.

Yams may be grated or shredded.

Combine onion, shredded yam, sausage, and basil in a slow cooker. Pour the eggs into the slow cooker after whisking them together.

Garlic powder, salt, and pepper are sprinkled on top of the dish. Add basil to the mix.

Cook for 8 hours on low with the lid off. The pie should be cut into wedges.

Stuffed Peppers is the name of the dish.

4 people Ingredients:

14 cup beef stock 1 pound ground meat 12 head cauliflower 1 carrot, chopped 4 peppers (bell) 1 chopped onion

Tomato paste (six ounces)

4 garlic cloves, minced

14 cup seasoning mix (Italian)

to taste with salt and pepper In a food processor, combine the carrots, cauliflower, garlic, and onion.

Pulse till the texture is fine.

Remove the tops of the peppers, remove the seeds, but leave the shell intact, and put aside.

Fill a bowl halfway with the vegetable mixture.

In a mixing dish, combine the meat, seasonings, and tomato paste. Salt & pepper to taste.

Blend until smooth.

Fill the bell peppers' hollows with the mixture.

Fill to the rim of the pepper with the mixture and place in the slow cooker.

Remove the tops of the bell peppers and replace them. Pour in the stock, cover, and simmer on low for 8 hours.

Gourmet Potatoes is the name of the dish.

4 people Ingredients: 2 pound of baby potatoes 1 tsp parsley (dry) olive oil, 2 tbsp

a teaspoon of dill

to taste with salt and pepper Clean the potatoes under running water and wipe dry.

Toss the potatoes in a basin with the olive oil, dill, and salt & pepper. Toss until everything is evenly covered.

Cook 4 hours on high, covered.

Place on a platter.

Serve with a parsley garnish.

2 servings Honeyed Walnuts Ingredients: cups walnuts

butter (tbsp)

14 cup of honey

1 tsp vanilla extract Ingredients: 1 tsp vanilla extract Directions:

Butter should be added to the slow cooker Set

until the butter has melted

Mix in the honey and vanilla extract. Stir in the walnuts to coat them.

Cook 2 hours on high, covered. Serve

1 container of pumpkin butter, 1 container of pumpkin butter, 1 container of pumpkin butter, 1 container of pumpkin butter, 1 15 oz pumpkin puree (optional)

honey (1/4 cup)

apple cider, 1/3 cup

a quarter cup of maple syrup

1 teaspoon pumpkin pie seasoning Directions: Combine all ingredients in a slow cooker.

Cover and cook on low for 4 hours.

4 Servings Title: Sweet Bananas

4 bananas (cut into thin pieces) 3

a tablespoon of honey

1 teaspoon of lemon juice 1 tsp cinnamon 1 tbsp coconut oil

1 teaspoon of cloves

nutmeg, 1 tsp In a slow cooker, combine the lemon juice, honey, and coconut oil.

COOK UNTIL THE KALE, GARLIC, AND LEEK ARE AROMATIC

spice sprinkling

Set the temperature to high and wait for the mixture to come together. Add bananas to the mix.

Cover and cook on low for 2 hours.

Roasted Beets is a recipe for roasted beets.

2 people

2 1 cup beets Ingredients

1 tablespoon honey

cinnamon (1 tsp)

1/3 cup liquid Directions: Combine all ingredients in a slow cooker.

Cook on low heat for 6 hours.

Sweet Potatoes is the name of a kind of potato. 4 people Ingredients:

4 big sweet potatoes, sliced into pieces

nutmeg, 1/8 teaspoon 1/8 teaspoon of cloves

a quarter teaspoon of cinnamon 2 tablespoons honey

1 cup unsweetened applesauce Sweet potatoes should be placed in a slow cooker. Add

except for honey, the remaining components Cook for 3 hours on low with the lid off.

Remove the slow cooker from the heat and place it on a platter.

Serve with honey drizzle

Stuffed Apples is a recipe for stuffed apples. 4 people 4 green apples, peeled and cored

4 tbsp coconut flakes

14 cup unsweetened sunbutter 12 cup heated coconut butter 2 tbsp cinnamon

nutmeg, 1 tsp

1 quart of liquid

1 teaspoon of salt Instructions: Core the apples but leave the bottoms intact.

Nutmeg, salt, cinnamon, coconut butter, and sunbutter should all be blended in a small basin.

Place the apples in the slow cooker.

Water should be poured.

Fill the apples with the butter mixture until they are completely full. Sprinkle

strew shredded coconut on top of the apples

Cover and cook on low for 3 hours.Butter should be added to the slow cooker Set

until the butter has melted

Mix in the honey and vanilla extract. Stir in the walnuts to coat them.

Cook 2 hours on high, covered. Serve

1 container of pumpkin butter, 1 container of pumpkin butter, 1 container of pumpkin butter, 1 container of pumpkin butter, 1 15 oz pumpkin puree (optional)

honey (1/4 cup)

apple cider, 1/3 cup

a quarter cup of maple syrup

1 teaspoon pumpkin pie seasoning Directions: Combine all ingredients in a slow cooker.

Cover and cook on low for 4 hours.

4 Servings Title: Sweet Bananas

4 bananas (cut into thin pieces) 3

a tablespoon of honey

1 teaspoon of lemon juice 1 tsp cinnamon 1 tbsp coconut oil

1 teaspoon of cloves

nutmeg, 1 tsp In a slow cooker, combine the lemon juice, honey, and coconut oil.

spice sprinkling

Set the temperature to high and wait for the mixture to come together. Add bananas to the mix.

Cover and cook on low for 2 hours.

Roasted Beets is a recipe for roasted beets.

2 people

2 1 cup beets Ingredients

1 tablespoon honey

cinnamon (1 tsp)

1/3 cup liquid Directions: Combine all ingredients in a slow cooker.

Cook on low heat for 6 hours.

Sweet Potatoes is the name of a kind of potato. 4 people Ingredients:

4 big sweet potatoes, sliced into pieces

nutmeg, 1/8 teaspoon 1/8 teaspoon of cloves

a quarter teaspoon of cinnamon 2 tablespoons honey

COOK UNTIL THE KALE, GARLIC, AND LEEK ARE AROMATIC

1 cup unsweetened applesauce Sweet potatoes should be placed in a slow cooker. Add

except for honey, the remaining components Cook for 3 hours on low with the lid off.

Remove the slow cooker from the heat and place it on a platter.

Serve with honey drizzle

Stuffed Apples is a recipe for stuffed apples. 4 people 4 green apples, peeled and cored

4 tbsp coconut flakes

14 cup unsweetened sunbutter 12 cup heated coconut butter 2 tbsp cinnamon

nutmeg, 1 tsp

1 quart of liquid

1 teaspoon of salt Instructions: Core the apples but leave the bottoms intact.

Nutmeg, salt, cinnamon, coconut butter, and sunbutter should all be blended in a small basin.

Place the apples in the slow cooker.

Water should be poured.

Fill the apples with the butter mixture until they are completely full. Sprinkle

strew shredded coconut on top of the apples

Cover and cook on low for 3 hours.